100 Ways to Lose Weight
Copyright © 2014 Leann Forst

The content of this book is for general instruction only. Each person's physical, emotional, and spiritual condition is unique. The teaching in this book is not intended to replace or interrupt the reader's relationship with a physician or other professional. Please consult your health coach or doctor for matters about your specific health and diet.

To contact the author, visit
www.groovybeets.com

Printed in the United States of America

ISBN-13:
978-1499724004

ISBN-10:
1499724004

Self-Help/Motivational and Inspirational

TABLE OF CONTENTS

PREFACE

I wasn't always a health coach. To put it mildly, I loved to eat, and I ate anything I wanted. My favorite was a large cheesy pizza, and I would eat the WHOLE thing in one sitting. I loved Buffalo wings, late-night hamburgers, potato skins, Chinese food... you name it. That's why my friends nicknamed me, 'The Feeder.' I'm not kidding.

(I'm going to tell you my story, so stick with me... you will see the relevance to you and the reason you chose to read this book.)

Fast forward to the age of 32 when I met and married my husband and began to try to have children: first, we had a miscarriage... ok, it could happen to anybody. Then we had our amazing little boy. However, when trying for our 2nd child, we had 2 more miscarriages. For anyone who has suffered through a miscarriage, you know what I'm talking about when I say 'it changes you.' It's not just a lost pregnancy; it's a lost child. My husband and I sought help from fertility specialist after fertility specialist; 5 in total. They kept giving me answers and advice that I did not want to hear, and I would not accept.

"Be happy with the one you have."

"It's just not in the cards for you."

'You are of advanced maternal age."

"You should go back on the pill to avoid any more heartbreak."

"You don't have any good eggs left."

Call me 'hard-headed, stubborn, persistent, determined or crazy'…. whatever it was; I KNEW that I was supposed to have another child. So, I stopped listening and started reading… everything I could get my hands on that had to do with health. I read about inflammation, food allergies, adrenal fatigue, the yeast connection, our food supply issues, genetically modified foods, pesticides, and on and on….

DING! DING! DING!

The light bulb went on as bright as it has ever been. There was a food connection to my health AND my unhealthy pregnancies.

So on the day that I 'went off the deep end,' as my husband puts it, I just got mad that no one - not my OB GYN, not my fertility specialists, not my family doctor, had told me that I should maybe take a look at what I was eating and clean up my diet to clean up my body and put it in the best possible position to have a healthy pregnancy. On that day, I threw out EVERYTHING in my pantry, my refrigerator, and my freezer.

3 months later, I was pregnant with my beautiful baby girl.

The stars began to align.

In that same year, my two-year-old son was sick with chronic asthma. Every 3 weeks, if he hadn't had a wheezing episode, I knew it was coming. When he was sick, it was for 10 days. It was cyclical. Again, our number was 5… we had been to 5 different asthma and allergy doctors with no relief. At the worst time, he was on 5 different medications. A visit to a holistic doctor gave us the simple advice that changed our lives forever.   Within months, he was asthma free and living life actively and without regular asthma medication and still is.

By now you might be asking, "what does this story have to do with WEIGHT LOSS?"

The answer is food.   Food is the connection to everything. And our food supply is not the same as it was 30 years ago when it was clean and nutritious.   Our food supply is in an alarming condition.   We are drowning in a chemically-laden, processed world, and it's killing us slowly.   Our pantries are full of processed boxed laboratory creations.   Artificial dyes are making our kids hyper and creating learning disabilities. Pesticides are now the number 3 cause of cancer behind smoking and every other environmental toxin put together. Genetically modified foods that are altered with the BT toxin are now clearly creating havoc with our digestive and immune systems.   Many dairy and livestock farming practices are in a shocking state of disgrace and disgust.   Animals are abused, shot up with antibiotics and scrunched into tiny living spaces. Food companies are adding chemicals into our food, and it's making us fat and sick.

It's no wonder virtually ALL of our disease rates including cancer, heart disease, diabetes, ADHD, allergies, asthma, and obesity - to name a few - are rising at unprecedented rates despite the fact that the United States spends more on healthcare than any other nation.

Maybe you are saying: "I don't have a disease, I just want to lose some weight."   "Still... what does disease have to do with weight loss?" The answer is inflammation.   It is now known that fat is linked to inflammation.   95% of diseases are now thought to be associated with inflammation.   Poor food quality causes inflammation which fuels fat cells to grow.

Did you know that the childhood obesity rate is now at a whopping 33%? The current generation of children is on track to living shorter lifespans than their parents. Shocking? Yes. Sad? Definitely. It's time to take our health back.

Despite what you have been told, losing weight is not about counting calories. Think about it, does it make sense that 500 calories are 500 calories whether it's a juicy steak, a bag of Cheetos or a green salad? NO. Your body does not process them the same way, and they all have different metabolic reactions within your body. If you are nourishing your body with healthy, whole foods, then you do not need to count calories. REALLY!

So what is this book going to do for you?

First, it's going to give you quick down and dirty easy tips, tricks, and transitions to switch to a real food way of eating. The idea is to 'crowd out' the bad food because you are eating so much good food that you are getting satisfied and full. No lengthy explanations, long chapters or medical mumbo jumbo, just straight to the point with the research to back it up. You can choose to move through the book one step at a time until you master it then move on to the next, you can jump around and try some that sound more appealing than others, or you can jump in with both feet and overhaul your life by incorporating as many changes as you can as fast as you can. It's up to you and how quickly you want to see change.

Second, by incorporating these changes you will become a slimmer you and by default, healthier. This is not a fad diet. This is not an off and on again diet. This is a change of the way you are living and eating so that you can change your life for good. By including some of these tips into your daily routine at your own pace, my promise to you is that your energy will improve, your mood will lift, you will easily shed pounds, and you will be healthier. The bonus is that by doing many of these small changes that make a big difference, you will start to incorporate healthier choices for you and change the path that your kids may be on. That is worth the cost of this book times 1000.

ABOUT THE AUTHOR

Leann holds a Master's degree from Drake University in Des Moines, Iowa and a Bachelor of Science from Upper Iowa University. Born and raised as an Iowa farm girl, she moved to Texas in 1998 where she met and married her husband. She had been in sales and marketing for 20 years until her life turned an abrupt corner when faced with challenging health issues for herself and her family that traditional medicine could not help.

As a die-hard researcher and determined mother, Leann improved her family's health and went on to become a Board Certified Holistic Health Practitioner and Food Toxin Expert studying over 100 dietary and healing theories at the Institute of Integrative Nutrition, the World's Largest Nutrition School.

Leann teaches moms to identify food toxins and triggers that are making their family sick. She also volunteers on her school district's School Health Advisory Committee so as to bring health initiatives to over 53 schools through nutrition and activity programs.

Please note: Leann is not a doctor, nutritionist or dietician. As a Board Certified Holistic Health Practitioner, helping people to meet their wellness goals, Leann is certified by the American Association of Drugless Practitioners. The information in this book is not intended to substitute for conventional medical advice, diagnosis or treatment; Leann encourages you to seek your healthcare provider's opinion. For holistic guidance, you may contact Leann at leann@groovybeets.com to set up a free health history consultation by phone.

Leann Forst owns GroovyBeets.com. It's based on research and evidence from leading experts in the field of natural heath and healing. The FTC requires full disclosure of relationships that Leann has between brands when writing about products. Brand and advertisers do not influence the content of Groovybeets.com because Leann chooses all content. Leann shares her opinion based on personal experience, education, and research and would never recommend a product that she would not use, has not used, or has personal experience with. Her goal is to share information with her readers so that they can make more informed decisions on creating a healthy family – because she was once there – without the knowledge to help herself or her child with asthma. Leann says, "I didn't make the connection between my food and my health. My wish is that you make this connection so that YOU can lead your best life."

GroovyBeets.com also gives back to the community by supporting school programs to teach kids healthy lifestyles.

information in this book is intended for informational purposes only and should not be considered professional advice.

INTRODUCTION

Obesity is a growing concern worldwide. The prevalence of obesity has risen dramatically in developed countries over the past 2 to 3 decades. Obesity has reached epidemic proportions in the United States with more than 20% of adults defined as clinically obese and an additional 30% identified as overweight. In 2013, 33% of children in the United States were overweight. Since overweight adolescents have a 70% chance of becoming overweight or obese adults (80% if even one parent is obese or overweight) the prognosis for the future health of Americans is declining. In American society, the immediate consequence of being overweight is social discrimination, often causing poor self-esteem and depression. Overweight or obese adults are also at risk for some chronic diseases, including heart disease, type 2 diabetes, high blood pressure, and some forms of cancer. Indeed, type 2 diabetes, previously considered an adult disease, has increased dramatically in children and adolescents along with the increase in obesity.

Change needs to happen. Food is our future.

CHAPTER 1
BEVERAGE STRATEGY

Many people don't give a second thought to what they drink throughout the day because they think since it's just liquid it must not have any real effect on their body, their health or their weight. I believe that making the small change in what you drink is one of the easiest changes to make. Check out the YouTube Video called "Pouring On The Pounds" to see how long it takes to walk off just one soda. Then think before you drink. Here are some ways to get started to drinking yourself skinny.

1. **Drink green tea** – it contains a compound called ECCG which promotes fat burning. One study noted a reduction in food intake in rats that were given a polyphenol, which is found in green tea. Another study concluded that green tea had heat-producing and calorie-burning properties beyond what can be explained by caffeine. When 31 healthy young men and women were given three servings of a beverage containing green tea catechins, caffeine, and calcium for three days, their 24-hour energy expenditure increased by 4.6%, according to the research from Lausanne University in Switzerland. Not too bad for doing nothing but drinking some tea.[1]

2. **Drink a cup of Java** – Caffeine stimulates your central nervous system, which regulates your heart rate. A Study published in the *American Journal of Clinical Nutrition* reported that the average metabolic rate of people that drank caffeinated coffee had a 16% higher metabolic rate than those who didn't.[2]

3. Drink 8 x 8 – Researchers at the University of Utah found that when volunteers drank eight 8 ounces of ice water per day, they had higher metabolic rates than those who only drank 4 glasses per day. Your body can burn calories when it works to heat the water to your core temperature. E. Wayne Askew, Ph.D., professor and director of the Division of Foods and Nutrition at the University of Utah College of Health, has found evidence that eight 8-oz. glasses of water a day, not only helps to maintain the body's hydration status but may bolster its metabolic rate as well, resulting in a more efficient burning of calories.[3]

4. Try fruit infused water instead of drinking fruit juice – Got a sweet tooth, but don't want the calories? A fruit infuser will give you the goodness of fruit, without the glycemic load of the pure juice. Consider it a watered down juice version with benefits. I like the Aquazinger from Brookstone. http://www.brookstone.com/aqua-zinger-flavored-water-maker

5. Replace your bagel with a nutrient dense smoothie – Use a high quality plant based protein powder, with a tablespoon of healthy fat such as almond butter, some blueberries or strawberries and a cup of your favorite non-dairy milk. When your diet is based on nutrient-dense foods, you will simultaneously flood your cells and tissues with protective substances and naturally guide your body to its ideal weight, with no hunger or feeling of deprivation. Nutrient-dense foods are rich in vitamins, minerals, phytochemicals, and antioxidants – and are low in calories. See Dr. Joel Fuhrman's food pyramid (resource is located in the bibliography) if you need some food ideas to get started.[4]

6. **Try this water alternative** – If you're bored with plain old water, try naturally-flavored seltzer — carbonated water with a shot of fruit flavor. It's completely calorie-free, fizzes like soda, and comes in fun flavors like green apple, cherry, pomegranate... even vanilla and white chocolate! And it's one of the "cleanest" drinks around — it doesn't contain sugar, artificial sweeteners, food dyes, or anything else. For sweetness and pizzazz, float a few fruit slices or frozen fruit cubes made with 100% juice in your glass.

CHAPTER 2
MEAL STRATEGY

Here's where we start getting into the nitty-gritty.   Who doesn't love food?   The best part about this section is that you don't have to starve yourself or count a single calorie, unlike what was once thought.   It's all about when, how, and what you eat.   It's about strategy.   These eating strategies have been proven to work.   The best part is that you can embrace ALL of them at once or one at a time.

7. **Aim for 30 grams of protein at every meal** – Protein helps to build more muscle and, even at rest, muscle burns more calories than fat says Dr. Donald Layman, Ph.D. professor of nutrition at the University of Illinois.   30 grams is approximately one turkey burger patty, one chicken breast or one cup low fat cottage cheese.   In a study published in *Nutrition Metabolism*, dieters who increased their protein intake to 30 percent of their diet ate nearly 450 fewer calories a day and lost about 11 pounds over the 12-week study without employing any other dietary measures.[5]

8. **Eat breakfast** – In a study published in the *American Journal of Epidemiology*, volunteers who skipped breakfast had 4 to 5 times the risk of obesity than those who ate breakfast.   The best breakfast is one with lean protein, complex carbs, and healthy fat.   Think oatmeal topped with walnuts and a cup of yogurt on the side.[6]

9. Add 2 tablespoons of ground flaxseed per day to your morning smoothie or oatmeal – Flaxseed is full of fiber to fill you up, keeping you from binging later on. Wellness expert Kathy Freston, the bestselling author of *Veganist* and *Quantum Wellness*, says 'one of the easiest things you can do to speed weight loss is to add two tablespoons of flaxseed into your daily regimen by sprinkling it into your morning oatmeal, adding it into a smoothie or mixing it into a salad. Flaxseed is low in carbohydrates and high in B vitamins, omega-3 fatty acids and fiber, which fills you up faster and keeps you satiated longer.' You can buy flaxseed in the health food section of the grocery store or a specialty store like GNC, and it should last for six weeks in the refrigerator.[7]

10. Eat dark green salad before dinner – According to Michelle Cardel, Ph.D., R.D.A, in a 2013 issue of *Academy Today*, eating a salad before a meal can reduce your caloric intake during the meal and over the course of the entire day. Eating a salad first may also help boost vegetable consumption by 23 percent, according to a study published in 2012 in the journal *Appetite*.[8]

11. Take your lunch to work – Dieters who eat out for lunch even once a week lose 5 fewer pounds on average according to *Journal of the Academy of Nutrition and Dietetics*.[9]

12. No carbohydrates after lunch – is one of the hardest rules to follow. But if you follow this one rule, you WILL lose weight says Bob Harper, a professional trainer from The Biggest Loser show.[10]

13. Don't eat after 6 p.m. – We've heard this one for a long time, after all, when was the last time your late night binge was a salad? Researchers from

Brigham Young University actually put the theory to the test, and the results showed that participants ate an average of 238 calories less per day, which led to half a pound of weight loss a week.[11]

14. **Drop some G-BOMBS** – The term coined by Dr. Joel Fuhrman, author of *Super Immunity*, stands for Greens, Beans, Onions, Mushrooms, Berries, and Seeds. These nutrient dense foods have powerful anti-cancer and anti-fat storage effects. These two work together because any food that protects against fat storage also protects against abnormal cell tissue or tumors. When you give your body nutrient dense foods, you naturally guide it to its ideal weight.[12]

15. **Eat 'lean and green' for dinner** – It works so well that the weight loss experts at Medifast Weight Control Centers trademarked the phrase. If you are aiming to lose a lot of weight fast, then this is a must. This gives you an excuse to spend less time in the kitchen. How hard is it to bake chicken and steam some broccoli? Add a LITTLE low, sugar teriyaki sauce or spicy brown mustard and you can instantly change up the taste. Add the chicken to a green salad the next night.[13]

16. **Eat four or five 400-calorie meals a day instead of 3 large meals** – This evens out your metabolism during the day. Tosca Reno, a leader in the Clean Eating movement, says that when you keep meals small – think the size of your palm – "your energy intake is spread throughout the day, and this will contribute to weight loss."[14]

17. **Snack on fermented foods** – such as pickles, kombucha, coconut yogurt, miso, tempeh, kimchi or sauerkraut. These probiotic powerhouses boost the good bacteria in your digestive tract which then can help heal health issues, like leaky gut and IBS, in

turn leading to weight loss, better skin, and boosted immunity. One of the reasons? "The gut is the largest part of our immune system," explains Drew Ramsey, MD, author of *The Happiness Diet* and *50 Shades of Kale*. So it matters what you put in it. "Sugar and refined carbohydrates cause damage, while fermented foods heal."[15]

18. **Choose organic** – Eating fresh produce is the best way to obtain the nutrients that support optimum health, but the pesticides used on many crops are a major health concern. By choosing organic foods, you can reap the health benefits of fruits and vegetables without exposing yourself and your family to potentially harmful chemicals. Pesticides present real health risks, particularly to children and those with health concerns. The toxicity most commonly associated with pesticides in animal studies includes disruption in the normal functioning of the nervous and endocrine system and increased risks of cancer. Researchers in Canada found in one study that the volunteers with the most pesticide chemicals stored in their fat cells were most at risk for thyroid dysfunction and mitochondrial damage. This damage can lead to weight gain. Can't afford to go all-organic? The following "Dirty Dozen Plus" (from the Environmental Working Group) had the highest pesticide load, making them the most important to buy or grow organic:

- Apples
- Strawberries
- Grapes
- Celery
- Peaches
- Spinach

- Sweet bell peppers
- Nectarines
- Cucumbers
- Cherry tomatoes
- Snap peas
- Potatoes
- Hot peppers
- Blueberries

Another easy rule of thumb: If you eat the skin, then go organic otherwise you are ingesting an average of 47 to 67 chemicals on EACH piece of fruit or veggie you eat... even after you wash it.[16]

19. **Try the Anti-Inflammatory Diet** – Reducing inflammation is the key to reducing fat, according to Dr. Weil, the revolutionary thinker behind the anti-inflammatory diet concept. The Anti-Inflammatory Diet is one that is designed to lower inflammation in the body. The Anti-Inflammatory Diet is based on a daily intake of 2,000 to 3,000 calories, depending on your gender, size, and activity level. About 40 to 50 percent of your calories will come from carbs, 30 percent from fat, and 20 to 30 percent from protein. Weil suggests striving for a mix of all three nutrients at each meal.[17]

20. **Use food combining** – Food combining is a secret to eating that enhances your digestion to give you energy and to help you lose weight and keep it off. According to Dr. Wayne Pickering, a naturopathic physician, and leader in food combining says that food combining is based on the idea that different foods should be eaten at different meals because they are digested and absorbed differently. Dr. Pickering lays out three basic commandments of eating that he recommends:

- No proteins and starches at the same meal, as they neutralize each other and prevent proper digestion of either food. To ensure proper digestion of each food, wait two hours after eating a starch before eating protein. And wait three hours after eating protein before eating starch.
- No fruits and vegetables at the same meal. According to Dr. Pickering, this is also why it's crucial not to eat dessert *after* a meal. When you do, it gets trapped in your stomach with all that other food, where it starts to rot, as it's not being chemically digested there. Therefore, eat fruit 30-60 minutes *before* dinner.
- Eat melon alone. Melons do not digest well with other foods and will frequently cause bloating and digestion issues unless consumed by itself.[18]

21. **Snack on nuts and seeds** – One of the country's leading nutrition scientists, Richard Mattes of Purdue, says that nuts have several good things going for them. For starters, even a small amount can make you feel full. Why do nuts appease the appetite so well? "They're high in protein, and protein is satiating," he said. "They're high in fiber, and fiber is satiating. They're rich in unsaturated fats, and there is some literature that suggests that it has satiety value. They're crunchy, and that would suggest just the mechanical aspect of chewing, which generates a satiety signal." Snacking on nuts makes it likely that you will eat less later in the same day, according to some research. That decrease in consumption can make up for many of the nuts' calories — as much as three-fourths of them, studies have shown. Nuts are also resistant to digestion, thanks to the tough walls of their cells. As much as one-fifth of the fat in nuts never gets absorbed by the

body, Dr. Mattes estimated in a 2008 paper published in *The Journal of Nutrition*.[19]

22. **Pack a snack bag always** – Some good snacks to have with you include whole grain crackers, small natural almond butter packets, apple slices, a wrapped boiled egg and yes, even a bit of dark chocolate. Don't forget your stainless steel water bottle with clean water. That way you don't splurge for the BPA-laden plastic water bottle that will mess up your hormones and hinder your weight loss efforts.[20]

23. **Eat more MUFAs** – Monounsaturated fatty acids, or MUFAs, help to decrease abdominal fat, according to the March 2007 *The Journal for Diabetes Care*. MUFAs are essential fats that are found in avocados, oils, olives, nuts, seeds, and dark chocolate. *The Flat Belly Diet*, by author Liz Vaccariello, suggests eating a small portion of MUFAs with every meal to achieve belly fat burning benefits. Serving suggestions include 1 tbsp. of oil, 1/4 cup of avocado, 10 almonds or other nuts, 10 olives or 1/4 cup of dark chocolate.[21]

24. **Eat at least 80 percent things that grow and no more than 20 percent things that walk** – A great tip from Lisa McRee, former Good Morning America co-host who lost 30 lbs.[22]

25. **Balance your thyroid with sea vegetables** – Thyroid health is essential for a smooth running metabolism. According to the *American Thyroid Association*, approximately 40% of the world's population remains at risk for iodine deficiency. Iodine is an element that is needed for the production of thyroid hormone. The body does not make iodine, so it is an essential part of your diet, without it, the body processes begin to slow down.

Hypothyroidism is linked to iodine deficiency and may cause weight gain in some individuals. To add more iodine to your diet with ease, try sprinkling your food with a shaker of sea vegetables. You can find it in any health food store in the spice or Japanese food aisle. Don't turn your nose up until you try it! It adds just a little salty flavor to your food, and your body will love you for it.[23]

26. **Add a purée to your favorite dish** – According to a study in the *American Journal of Clinical Nutrition*, researchers from Penn State gave 20 men and 21 women casseroles made with varying amounts of purée — a strategy popularized by the cookbook author Jessica Seinfeld, who has encouraged parents to sneak vegetables into foods like spaghetti.

But in the Penn State study, the goal wasn't to trick people into eating vegetables. Adding the purée bulked up the dish and resulted in fewer calories per serving. When they were served the casseroles made with puréed vegetables, they ate 200 to 350 fewer calories a meal.[24]

27. **Try Thai** – Some studies have shown that very spicy foods, such as Thai, can increase metabolism by about 20% for about 30 minutes. A study in 2003 evaluated 10 Thai women and their glucose response after a glucose drink and their metabolic rate before and after a spicy Thai dish. The result was an immediate increase of 20% in their metabolic rate within a few minutes of eating.[25]

28. **Use a spritzer** – for salad dressings instead of pouring it on. Saving calories are better than counting calories.

CHAPTER 3
SUPPLEMENT STRATEGY

Supplements can be a great way to give your weight loss efforts a jump start.   And while all of the supplements discussed in this chapter are generally recognized as safe, it's important that you use good judgment and discuss them with your health practitioner if you are on medications.   It's important to be eating real food before adding in a supplement program. Otherwise, it's just money down the drain because you will be sabotaging your efforts.

29. **Replace your hum-drum multi-vitamin with one a high quality one that contains chlorella** – According to the *Science of Eating*, chlorella is an astounding package of complete nutrition and benefits weight loss in several different ways. It is super low in calories but is a complete food nutritionally, so ingesting it can dramatically help to eliminate food cravings.   This happens because people feel hungry when the body is really craving nourishment due to poor nutrition.   Plus, when we replace nutritionally empty foods with powerful superfoods like chlorella, the body tends to crave less junk food because it feels more nourished. Chlorella balances your endocrine system and creates an environment in the body that favors weight loss.   Chlorella promotes the production of healthy flora throughout the digestive system.   This is essential for good digestion and overall health, and makes chlorella effective for fighting candida and yeast overgrowth.   One Japanese study showed

that chlorella reduces body fat percentages, due to its ability to aid fat metabolism and improve insulin sensitivity.[26]

30. Take a probiotic supplement in the morning – There are over 400 types of healthy bacterial organisms in our digestive tract. These organisms are tasked with the maintenance of our health. When the balance between good and bad bacteria gets out of whack, the result is a bloated tummy. According to a study by the *British Journal of Nutrition*, researchers from Laval University in Quebec instructed 125 overweight women to follow a 12-week weight loss diet, followed by a 12-week maintenance period. Half of the participants also swallowed probiotic pills every day, and the other half got placebo pills. What happened? After the 12-week weight loss period, the women who took the probiotic pills had lost 9.7 pounds on average, while the women who took the placebos only lost 5.7 pounds. And then, after the 12-week maintenance period, the women who took the placebo pills maintained a stable weight, but the probiotics group continued to slim down, losing 1.8 more pounds, on average. By the study's end, the women in the probiotics group also had less of the intestinal bacteria related to obesity. Don't take on an empty stomach or with coffee; the acidity will cancel the benefit.[27]

31. High quality essential fatty acid supplement – EFAs accelerate fat burning. In the presence of essential fatty acids, cells burn greater amounts of oxygen. The more oxygen carried to the cells, the faster the body fat is burned. A Harvard School of Public Health report states: "Fats are also biologically active molecules that can influence how muscles respond to insulin's "open up for sugar" signal; different types of fats can also fire up or cool down inflammation." Does the thought of fish oil make you gag? Try Barlean's brand of flavored fish oil. My family loves the strawberry swirl flavor.[28]

32. **Comprehensive multi-mineral at night** – Some researchers believe that overweight people have lowered immunity. This could be from deficiencies of vitamins and minerals, especially the antioxidants. According to a study done in Poland, overweight people may not be reaping antioxidant benefits. Researchers at the National Institute of Food and Nutrition in Warsaw studied 102 overweight women and found that the women had significantly lower levels of the antioxidant vitamins C and E, as well as of vitamin A, and a higher prevalence of overall vitamin deficiency than those of normal weight. These deficiencies are at least partially responsible for depressing immunity in overweight individuals, leaving them more susceptible to cancer and infectious illness, said some researchers. And because of abnormal hormone activity, overweight people may also have a greater need for antioxidants than individuals who are not overweight.[29]

A good multi-mineral product includes choline and inositol that work together to metabolize fat, iodine that stimulates your thyroid, chromium which processes carbs and reduces hunger pangs. Take it at night to help sleep and also to avoid it interfering with your vitamins.

33. **Vitamin D** – *Medical News Today* reported that there is a link between Vitamin D levels and successful weight loss. Also, according to Dr. Mercola, a new study of more than 4,600 women aged 65 and older shows that having low vitamin D levels can contribute to mild weight gain. Previous research has already shown that obese individuals tend to have low vitamin D levels. Women who had

insufficient levels of vitamin D gained about two pounds more compared to those with adequate blood levels of vitamin D during the 4.5-year long study. Those with insufficient levels also weighed more at the outset of the study.[30]

34. **Complex vitamin B** – Take in the morning to keep your metabolism running. Vitamin B Complex is a group of eleven vitamins that work together. Some of the B vitamins that aid in weight loss are B6 (pyridoxine), B5 (pantothenic acid), and B2 (riboflavin). Vitamin B6 helps the pancreas to produce enzymes that aid in digestion. Proper digestion will make one feel full longer, thus resulting in weight loss, Vitamin B5 also aids in digestion and helps to break down fat and carbohydrates, thus giving more energy and boosting one's metabolism, which also helps in weight loss. Vitamin B2 aids in weight loss by releasing the unused energy in the body and preventing unused energy from turning into fat. Some of the best sources of vitamin B are bananas, potatoes, whole grains, beans, lentils, and chili peppers.[31]

35. **Increase your vitamin C** – This helps to turn glucose into energy instead of being stored in your body as fat. Aim for 400 to 500 mg of C and 800 mg of D a day. According to The National Center for Biotechnology Information, which advances science and health by providing access to biomedical and genomic information, vitamin C status is inversely related to body mass. Individuals with adequate vitamin C status oxidize 30% more fat during a moderate exercise more than people with low vitamin C status; thus, vitamin C depleted individuals may be more resistant to fat mass loss.[32]

36. **CoQ10** – Coenzyme Q-10, also called ubiquinone, is a powerful antioxidant/anti-inflammatory with many benefits for treating and preventing obesity. It acts similarly to acetyl L-carnitine in that it assists in energy production within the mitochondria. CoQ10 enhances the metabolism, giving us greater energy and endurance, a greater ability to lose body fat, preventing the energy decline seen in aging cells. CoQ10 also maximizes the burning of foods for fuel, helping to normalize fats in our blood.[33]

37. **Glutamine** – According to the Muscle & Fitness article, 'The Ten Supps You Can't Live Without' by Jim Stoppani, glutamine boosts metabolism and fat burning. Not only does it increase fat burning when taken before and during exercise, but it also boosts your resting metabolic rate.[34]

38. **Vanadium** – This is now showing promise as a treatment to control blood glucose levels and reduce weight. There is, of course, a connection between insulin utilization and weight control, which is why compounds that control blood glucose (such as vanadium) are of interest to those trying to reduce their weight and type II diabetics. Optimal insulin utilization is a key factor in reducing fatty deposits in the midsection, commonly known as belly fat.[35]

39. **CLA** – CLA stands for Conjugated Linoleic Acid, which has been shown to reduce fat and increase lean body mass and has powerful anti-inflammatory activity. It decreases fat, especially in the area of the stomach and helps to block the absorption of fat into the fat cells. CLA works by facilitating the process by which your cells release fat.[36]

40. **Coconut oil** – This is a fat that can make you thin. Although we hear a lot about using olive oil, coconut oil provides MCTs, which have been shown

to boost your metabolism and help your body to burn fat more efficiently. One study in the journal *Lipids*, for example, showed that women who consumed about two tablespoons of coconut oil daily for 12 weeks reduced their belly fat and did not gain weight.[37]

41. **African mango** – Also called Irvingia gabonesis. There have been several studies conducted, which concluded that Irvingia gabonesis helps in both weight loss and percentage body fat loss. For instance, in a 2009 study in *Lipids in Health and Disease*, researchers found that participants who took African mango every day for 10 weeks experienced significant improvements in body weight, body fat, waist size, cholesterol levels, blood sugar levels, and levels of C-reactive protein (a marker of inflammation). The study involved 102 healthy overweight or obese people; half of the participants received African mango, while the other half were given a placebo.[38]

42. **Green coffee bean extract** – According to a Fox News article, one clinical study published in the scientific French review *Phytothérapie,* demonstrated fat-reducing effects of a green (non-roasted) coffee bean extract. One group of volunteers was given 400 mg of a decaffeinated green coffee extract daily, and the second group received a placebo. After 60 days of supplementation, participants who received the green coffee extract had lost 5.7 percent of their initial weight. By contrast, the group that received a placebo had lost 2.8 percent of their initial weight.[39]

43. **Alpha lipoic acid (ALA)** – *Life Extension Magazine* reports that lipoic acid has beneficial effects on the forces that cause us to gain weight and store excess fat. It works on brain areas to reduce appetite, food

intake, and body weight. Even in people who are only overweight (not yet obese), lipoic acid reduced body weight by 8% while shrinking waist size by more than 2 inches. In patients who are already obese, there was a 9% loss of weight and a decrease in waist size of more than 3 inches.[40]

44. Maitake mushroom D-Fraction – According to Dr. Nicholas Perricone, a board-certified dermatologist, world renowned healthy aging expert, award winning inventor, educator, and philanthropist, animal studies have shown that including maitake in your routine diet can reduce weight gain, not only because of its high–fiber, low-calorie quality, but because maitake also helps to boost metabolism rates.

Beta glucan is thought to be the source of maitake's ability to help:

- Control blood sugar by enhancing insulin sensitivity.
- Decrease your risk of cardiovascular disease and diabetes.
- Increase weight loss, especially around the abdomen.

Dr. Perricone recommends taking 1 caplet 3X a day between meals.[41]

CHAPTER 4
SWAP

I love swaps because it's a win-win… you still get to eat delicious food except you are swapping them for a healthier version. Anytime you can increase your nutrients and decrease nutrient-void food, your body will love you for it. Here are some of my favorite swaps that will trim you down in no time.

45. **Swap out cow's milk and replace with coconut milk, almond milk** – Even if you drink organic cow's milk, the cow's that provide the milk are still milked an average of 300 times a year. Much of that time, they are pregnant which means all those extra pregnancy hormones are going directly into your milk, messing up your hormones. According to Dr. Justin Butler's article in *Viva! Health*, a registered charity set up to monitor and explain the increasing amount of scientific research linking diet to health, all cow's milk, whether organic or non-organic, contains hormones and growth factors. It is, after all, baby food designed to help a newborn animal grow and the reason why growth factors are implicated in certain cancers.

All cow's milk contains:

- Hormones and growth factors – linked to cancers such as breast and prostate.
- Saturated animal fat – linked to obesity, type 2 diabetes, heart disease, and stroke.
- Casein – the milk protein linked to childhood allergies and type 1 diabetes in some children.

- Lactose – the sugar in milk is linked to ovarian cancer and responsible for the uncomfortable symptoms of lactose intolerance.[42]

46. **Swap out cow's milk yogurt and replace with coconut yogurt** – If you haven't tried these, you are missing out. My son loves them, and he is the ULTIMATE picky eater. Top with berries and you have a great healthy dessert that won't break your belt. Much of the saturated fat in coconut yogurt is in the form of medium-chain triglycerides, which can help to control weight, reduce the risk of atherosclerosis and boost immunity, according to a 2013 article in *Nutrition Review*.[43]

47. **Swap out cow's milk cheese and replace with goat cheese** – For example, 1 oz. of goat's cheese feta contains just 75 calories and 6 g of fat, while an ounce of cow's milk cheddar contains 114 calories and 9 g of fat. Fresh goat cheese and feta contain a fatty acid that helps you feel full and burn more fat. Look for cheeses labeled "grass-fed," as those will have the highest content of this healthy fat.[44]

48. **Swap out your bread and try Ezekiel bread** – Not only is Ezekiel bread made from sprouted whole grains and contain vital nutrients, but there is no added sugar… and we know what sugar does to our waistline. One study found that eating sprouted grain bread reduced the blood sugar response and increased the glucagon response when compared to eating unsprouted bread, 11-grain, 12-grain, white, or sourdough.[45]

49. **Swap out salted nuts and replace with unsalted nuts** – Excess salt means bloating and that can mimic weight gain in the respect that you may not be able to button up your jeans. Less salt, less

bloat. Salt will not stop weight loss, but it can stall it. Sodium makes your body retain water. When you eat too much salt, you may see the scale go up a few pounds. Conversely, when you significantly reduce salt intake, you'll lose a few pounds as your body expels the water it was retaining. The weight you lose, however, is regained once you resume eating foods with salt.[46]

50. **Swap out white rice chips and replace with brown rice chips** – When it comes to keeping your weight down, a new study by Harvard researchers suggests that the quality of your food matters more than its calorie count. In the most comprehensive and detailed study of its kind, researchers have figured out exactly how much weight gain is associated with the consumption of certain foods.

The worst offenders were potato chips, which led to more weight gain per serving than any other food. For each extra serving of potato chips eaten in a day, for instance, people gained 1.69 lbs. every four years. Among the other extra-fattening foods, the study highlighted: potatoes. baked, boiled, mashed or French fried, each extra serving of potatoes was associated with an average 1.28-lb. weight gain.[47]

51. **Swap out dairy based dips and replace with hummus** – Hummus is made out of chickpeas, which give you fiber, and fill you up more. People who regularly eat hummus tend to have smaller waists and healthier diets overall, a new study in the *Journal of Nutrition & Food Sciences* found. The researchers pulled data about chickpea and hummus consumption from the National Health and Nutrition Examination Survey and found that hummus eaters take in 52 percent more fiber, 13 percent more good-for-you polyunsaturated fats, and 20 percent less sugar than non-consumers. Plus, people who eat the

chickpea-based dip are healthier eaters overall, packing in more servings of fruit, dark green veggies, and whole grains per day.

Hummus eaters' waists are, on average, eight percent smaller than the waists of people who don't eat the dip, the study found. They also tend to weigh less, even though they take in no fewer calories overall.[48]

52. **Swap out white pasta for whole grain pasta** – White pasta lacks fiber, vitamins, and minerals. Emerging evidence suggests that whole grain intake may contribute to achieving and maintaining a healthy weight. Studies show that people who include whole grain as part of a healthful diet are less likely to gain weight over time. Eating a diet high in whole grains is associated with lower body mass index and weight, smaller waist circumference, and reduced risk of being overweight. People who consume more whole grains are likely to have healthier lifestyles.[49]

53. **Swap out oil when you bake and replace with applesauce** – In most baking recipes, you can swap out any oil on a 1 to 1 measurement with applesauce and get sweet results. Cut the fat while adding nutrients. Generally, the applesauce for oil substitution works best in bread, muffin, and cake recipes. By replacing the oil, you are removing unhealthy fats. Use natural applesauce to eliminate added sugar, as well.[50]

54. **Swap out white baked potatoes and replace with baked sweet potatoes** – Sweet potatoes are a delicious member of the dark orange vegetable family, which lead the pack in vitamin A content. Substitute a baked sweet potato (also loaded with vitamin C, calcium, and potassium) for a baked white potato. And before you add butter or sugar,

taste the sweetness that develops when a sweet potato is cooked -- and think of all the calories you can save over that loaded baked potato. "Sweet potatoes are a great source of dietary fiber, which helps to reduce blood sugar and insulin spikes, ultimately reducing belly fat," explains Shana Maleeff a dietitian and fitness professional in New York City.[51]

55. **Swap out regular hamburger and replace with bison burger** – Bison, also known as buffalo has been making a comeback over the last few decades. Bison meat, in most cases, is free of steroids, hormones, and antibiotics and is lower in fat, cholesterol, and calories than beef, pork, and even skinless chicken. Since Bison are more resistant to disease than cattle, there is no need for antibiotic feed. Bison is typically raised in a more natural environment than our current meat production system, so the Bison meat you buy comes without the hormones used to make cows grow fast and fat. Bison is also higher in iron and vitamin B12 than beef. Despite all these differences, Bison is very similar to beef in flavor and texture.

According to the USDA, a grass-fed, three-ounce bison patty has 152 calories and seven grams of fat. That's less than a broiled, 90 percent lean beef burger, which averages 184 calories and 10 grams of fat. It's even less than a broiled, 93 percent lean turkey burger, which averages 176 calories and 10 grams of fat. Most ground bison is at least 90 percent lean.[52]

56. **Swap out red meat in any dish and replace with ground turkey or better, chopped mushrooms** – Mushrooms are neither a fruit nor a vegetable but can be an excellent addition to your weight loss plan. According to Dr. Oz, if you're trying to lose

weight, then substituting Crimini mushrooms for meat will cut the fat without losing taste. The high-fiber mushroom mixture works well for any meat-based dish – tacos, meat sauce, hamburgers, and more. In addition, according to sports nutritionist, Dr. John Berardi on the *Muscle and Strength* website, the body uses more energy to digest protein than it does fat or carbohydrate, leading to faster weight loss. The type of meat you pick when dieting is important, as the calorie and fat content can vary greatly from one meat to the next.[53]

57. **Swap out sour cream in recipes and replace with Greek yogurt** – Can't live without sour cream on your next taco or baked potato? Or maybe you are a blood type B or AB that can handle a little dairy. Then don't go for the high fat sour cream, instead, try plain fat free Greek Yogurt. Greek Yogurt typically contains more protein and less lactose than sour cream or regular yogurt. So, even dairy intolerant people can dabble in a little Greek Yogurt now and then. Greek yogurt substitutes well for sour cream because their consistencies are similar. This means that when a cookie recipe calls for a cup of sour cream, a cup of Greek yogurt can be substituted. Yogurt specifically has been studied as a calcium-rich food that helps to burn fat and promotes weight loss. A University of Tennessee study in 2005 shows that dieters who ate three servings of yogurt a day lost 22% more weight and 61% more body fat than those who only cut calories. Those that lost the most weight were able to protect their lean muscle mass, which is critical when dieting because the muscle mass is essential for maintaining a high metabolism.[54]

58. **Swap out white rice and replace with quinoa** – Quinoa seeds are rich in essential amino acids and vitamins such as magnesium and calcium. Quinoa is

also high in iron and vitamin B 12. Both iron and vitamin B 12 are essential for energy production and weight loss. If you are deficient in B vitamins, it can slow down your weight loss because your body won't be able to synthesize nutrients as efficiently. Quinoa has the perfect balance of all nine amino acids essential for human nutrition. This type of complete protein is rarely found in plant foods, though common in meats. Quinoa also offers a healthy dose of fiber and iron. There are 111 calories in each 1/2-cup of cooked quinoa.[55]

59. **Swap out dairy butter and replace with coconut butter** – Baking with a healthier fat tends to make baked goods a little dryer, so you'll need to add a bit more of a moist ingredient such as fruit puree or oil. Coconut butter packs a ton of benefits: It's rich in lauric acid, which boosts immunity and destroys harmful bacteria, viruses, and fungi. It actually boosts your metabolism, which aids in weight loss and increases energy levels. It's packed with healthy fats, so you feel full longer.[56]

60. **Swap out regular frozen pizza and replace with whole grain pizza and swap out thick crust and replace with thin crust** – Pizza can have a wide range of calories – from relatively low to quite high. On average you'll save about 28 percent of the calories if you choose thin crust pizza over regular crust. Here are some nutrition and calorie facts from the USDA National Nutrient Database.[57]

The difference between slices may not seem like a lot but who can eat JUST ONE? See below for comparisons.

Frozen Pizza Calories and Nutrition Facts (per pizza slice)

Type of Pizza	Calories (kcal)	Weight (g)	Nutrition Facts				
			Fat (g)	Cholesterol (mg)	Sodium (mg)	Carbs (g)	Protein (g)
DiGiorno Frozen Pizza (1 slice = 1/4 pizza pie)							
cheese topping, cheese stuffed crust	458	164	19	46	1,322	49	22
cheese topping, rising crust	468	183	16	27	1,274	58	23
cheese topping, thin crispy crust	398	161	16	34	815	43	21
pepperoni topping, cheese stuffed crust	499	179	21	43	1,348	53	25
pepperoni topping, rising crust	549	207	21	37	1,538	64	26
pepperoni topping, thin crispy crust	410	145	19	41	961	42	19
supreme topping, rising crust	579	227	24	43	1,616	63	27
supreme topping, thin crispy crust	395	155	17	31	860	43	18
Kashi Frozen Pizza (1 slice = 1/3 pizza pie)							
Basil Pesto	240	113	9	14	593	27	14
Margherita	260	113	9	19	633	29	14
Mediterranean	277	120	9	14	637	37	15
Mushroom Trio & Spinach	251	113	9	26	663	28	14

26

Frozen Pizza Calories and Nutrition Facts (per pizza slice)

Type of Pizza	Calories (kcal)	Weight (g)	Nutrition Facts				
			Fat (g)	Cholesterol (mg)	Sodium (mg)	Carbs (g)	Protein (g)
Roasted Vegetable	260	116	10	19	633	28	15

Typical Frozen Pizza (1 slice = 1/4 pizza pie)

Type of Pizza	Calories (kcal)	Weight (g)	Fat (g)	Cholesterol (mg)	Sodium (mg)	Carbs (g)	Protein (g)
cheese topping, regular crust	488	182	22	25	814	53	19
cheese topping, rising crust	543	209	18	33	1,162	69	26
meat and vegetable topping, regular crust	491	178	26	28	988	45	20
meat & vegetable topping, rising crust	691	255	30	48	1,632	73	32
pepperoni topping, regular crust	592	200	30	30	1,236	57	22

61. **Swap out jelly with added sugar and replace with real fruit jelly with no added sugar** – This is a no-brainer. Many jellies are sweetened with everything from corn syrup to fruit juice concentrate to artificial sweeteners. Just don't forget to read the labels.

62. **Swap out high sugar peanut butter and replace with almond butter or cashew butter** – Check the label on your favorite peanut butter for added sugar. Big brands add a trivial 1 or 2 grams of sugar to the 1 or 2 grams that occur naturally in the peanuts. It's no big deal. But these days, "artisan" varieties can hit 9 grams of sugar per serving with 7 of them being added. That's 1½ of the six-teaspoon daily added sugar limit for women or the nine-teaspoon max for men. Some brands have enough sugar to displace a gram or two of protein. Not to mention that some peanuts have been found to have a fungus called aflatoxin. Who needs that? To be safe, switch to a better nut butter.[58]

63. **Swap out products that are "made with whole grains and replace with products that are 100 percent whole grain** – When a label says "made with whole grains" it typically means "made with mostly white flour." It's a marketing ploy. BONUS HEALTH TIP: Look for 'Gluten-Free Whole Grain' bread products. Gluten Free Diets are all the rage right now BUT just looking for "gluten free" may mean that the product has other less healthy ingredients like tapioca, which has little nutritional value and will make you fat. The best solution is to buy products that are gluten free AND whole grain such as buckwheat waffles, quinoa rice, and brown rice tortillas. They taste good too! Again, a diet rich in whole grains may help fight

your belly bulge while lowering the risk of heart disease.

If you are looking for more proof, a study in the *American Journal of Clinical Nutrition* shows that people who followed a weight loss program incorporating whole-grain bread, cereals, and other foods lost more body fat from the abdominal area than those who ate only refined grains like white bread and rice.[59]

64. **Swap out sugar and replace with honey** – The more of the white processed stuff you can cut out, the better your weight and health. Honey is still a sweetener, but at least you get the health benefits with it. Aren't all sugars the same? No, your body processes whole food, natural sugar such as honey differently than white processed table sugar. Honey contains 22 amino acids, which play an essential role in metabolism. As your metabolism increases, you burn more calories and increased energy levels. Sugar is made of 50 percent glucose and 50 percent fructose, the sugar typically found in fruits, and is broken down very easily, leading to a surge of blood glucose. What your body doesn't use right away gets stored as fat. Honey is also made mostly of sugar, but it's only about 30 percent glucose and less than 40 percent fructose. And there are also about 20 other sugars in the mix, many of which are much more complex, and dextrin, a type of starchy fiber. This means that your body expends more energy to break it all down to glucose. Therefore, you end up accumulating fewer calories from it.[60]

65. **Swap out white flour for baking and replace with whole grain, gluten free flour** – Personally, I like coconut flour. Coconut flour is high in fiber and can be a part of a healthy weight loss plan because it will give you a feeling of fullness. There are wide

variety of gluten-free, whole grain flours to choose from. Try a few for different recipes and see which one you prefer. Many websites provide conversion information for recipes originally created with white flour in mind. Check out the Gluten-Free Goddess for more information.

(http://glutenfreegoddess.blogspot.com/). [61]

66. **Swap out ice cream and replace with blended frozen bananas for 'ice cream'** – Try this. Freeze 3 ripe bananas then blend them with a squirt of honey and a splash of coconut or almond milk. Then smack your lips and say "Yum!" You will never need to eat regular ice cream again.[62]

67. **Swap out mayo and replace with mustard** – Spoon 5 teaspoons into any meal and, a couple of hours later, your fat burning will have increased by up to 20%. "The metabolism-boosting effects are thanks to chemical 'isothiocyanates' found in mustard, which dilates blood vessels and increases levels of the fat-burning hormone ephedrine," explains Jeya Henry, professor of human nutrition at Oxford Brookes University.[63]

68. **Swap out any pasta and replace with spaghetti squash** – Dr. Jonny Bowden, Ph.D. and Clinical Nutrition Specialist, and author of *The 150 Healthiest Foods on Earth*, says that there are two types of squash, summer squash and winter squash, and both offer specific advantages. Dr. Bowden reports that summer squash is good for weight loss because it is the lower of the two in calories. Spaghetti squash is a type of summer squash that is a particularly good diet food. One cup of spaghetti squash has only 42 calories and contains moderate amounts of potassium and vitamin A. It also has 2.2

grams of dietary fiber that can help to curb your appetite.[64]

69. **Swap out meat in most recipes and replace with tofu** – According to Weight Watchers, tofu adds a "wonderful creamy taste without all the fat." People following vegetarian diets commonly eat tofu. According to a review published in a 2011 edition of *Cancer Management and Research*, vegetarians weigh 3 to 20 percent less and have lower obesity rates than people who eat meat.[65]

70. **Swap out all cow's milk products** – I know, I know, you can't give up your cheese! But if you haven't tried cutting it before, I recommend it to every person who is seeking to lose weight OR battle a chronic illness. It contains lactose, which is sugar. Lactose intolerances can lead to bloating," says Robynne Chutkan, M.D. of the Digestive Center for Women in Chevy Chase, MD. If that isn't enough, cow's milk causes the body to produce mucus, especially in the gastro-intestinal tract. Cancer feeds on mucus. Think of a pond with green scum on the top. It's a place for bacteria to grow. By cutting off milk and substituting with non-dairy milk, cancer cells will starve.

So next time you reach for that tall glass of cow's milk, try coconut or almond milk. Replace cow's cheese with non-dairy cheese or goat cheese. Replace regular yogurt with coconut yogurt. Replace butter with coconut butter.[66]

71. **Swap out standard salad dressings and replace with balsamic vinegar** – One of the best ways balsamic vinegar can help you lose weight is by providing flavor without many calories. For example, a tablespoon of balsamic vinaigrette salad dressing contains a mere 43 calories. The same

amount of creamy ranch salad dressing contains at least 73 calories, nearly twice that of the balsamic vinaigrette. The book *The Healing Powers of Vinegar* discusses the effects of acetic acid, an essential compound found in balsamic vinegar and other varieties. Acetic acid helps to slow the absorption of carbohydrate foods as they are broken down in the body, helping to balance your blood sugar levels and reduce hunger. It also improves fat breakdown for more energy.[67]

CHAPTER 5
ADD

By now you have learned that losing weight is about strategy. What better strategy than ADDING certain foods to help you increase metabolism? Just by adding in these fat fighting foods and crowding out fat magnets, you can shave pounds, boost your energy, and stay full all day long.

72. **Add turmeric on your eggs, veggies or in your soups** – Curcumin, the compound in turmeric spice, is known for its anti-inflammatory properties and inflammation is the cornerstone of most chronic diseases, including obesity. It also reduces the formation of fat tissue by suppressing the blood vessels needed to form it. Research in the *European Journal of Nutrition* suggests that curcumin may be useful for the treatment and prevention of obesity-related chronic diseases, as the interactions of curcumin with several signal transduction pathways also reverse insulin resistance, hyperglycemia, hyperlipidemia, and other inflammatory symptoms associated with obesity and metabolic disorders.[68]

73. **Add organic edamame** – which is great for a protein snack. Protein slows the emptying of food from the stomach so that hunger does not return as soon after a meal. One cup of edamame, or boiled soybeans, contains 17 grams of protein, 8 grams of fiber, and 189 calories. A perfect snack all by itself! Serve hot or cold, season with salt, and enjoy. "It remains prudent to recommend soy in a heart-

healthy diet because of its nutritional value and as a healthy substitute for protein sources that are higher in saturated fat and cholesterol," says Pennsylvania State University nutrition researcher Penny Kris-Etherton, Ph.D., RD.[69]

74. Add prebiotic foods to nourish the probiotic foods – Barely ripe bananas, artichokes, asparagus, oatmeal, brown rice, and quinoa. Prebiotics are better than probiotics when it comes to weight loss and burning abdominal fat, according to some researchers. The findings, published in the *Journal of Functional Foods*, suggest that prebiotic fiber may help to prevent intestinal fat absorption and could be an effective weight loss tool. "Normally we digest all the food and absorb all the calories," said study researcher Peter Jones of the University of Manitoba in Canada. "We think the prebiotic fiber interfered with the absorption of those calories, so that more calories went out the tailpipe and there were fewer calories to pack on abdominal fat."[70]

75. Add apples and pears – Apples contain a fiber called pectin. According to the *Huffington Post*, researchers at UCLA showed that by swapping in pectin for regular fiber, they could double the time it took subjects' stomachs to empty from about 1 hour to 2 hours, which meant subjects felt full that much longer. And in another study published in the journal *Nutrition*, scientists found that instructing participants to eat an apple or a pear before meals resulted in significant weight loss.[71]

76. Add grapefruit – Ever tried the grapefruit diet? Turns out there may be some good research to back up grapefruit's reputation as a fat fighter. In a 2004 study at the Scripps Clinic in La Jolla, California, researchers investigated the effect of grapefruit on weight loss and found that eating half a grapefruit before a meal can actually help people drop weight, while also improving insulin resistance. The researchers studied the effect of grapefruit capsules, grapefruit juice, and real grapefruit. All three seemed to help, but the folks eating the real grapefruit got the best results. As an added benefit, grapefruit contains cancer-fighting compounds like liminoids and lycopene, and red grapefruit has been shown to help lower triglycerides. And half a grapefruit has only 39 calories.[72]

77. **Add spinach and kale** – Scientists at Lund University in Sweden have found that a spinach extract containing green leaf membranes called thylakoids curbed food cravings by 95 percent and boost weight loss by 43 percent. "Our analyses show that having a green drink containing thylakoids before breakfast reduces cravings and keeps you feeling more satisfied all day," says Charlotte Erlanson-Albertsson, Professor of Medicine and Physiological Chemistry at Lund University.[73]

78. **Add cruciferous vegetables** – According to Ori Hofmekler, author of *The Warrior Diet*, an imbalance in estrogen metabolism can cause your body to store more fat. Furthermore, it can also lead to estrogen-related diseases, such as breast cancer. An imbalance in estrogen metabolism is commonly associated with a diet low in vegetables. Symptoms of estrogen imbalance include: Inability to lose stubborn abdominal fat, reduced libido, chronic fatigue, and a reduction in the ability to tolerate stress. Hofmekler explains that estrogenic chemicals may be found in the diet in foods such as meat, beer, fruit, and vegetables treated with pesticides, soy foods, and artificial sweeteners. Cruciferous vegetables contain a large amount of

diindolymethane, a compound that can restore the balance of your estrogen metabolites.[74]

79. **Add buckwheat** – According to Dr. Perricone, the specific characteristics of buckwheat proteins, and the relative proportions of its amino acids make buckwheat the unsurpassed cholesterol-lowering food studied to date. Its protein characteristics also enhance buckwheat's ability to reduce and stabilize blood sugar levels following meals—a key factor in preventing diabetes and obesity. Additionally, like the widely prescribed "ACE" hypertension drugs, buckwheat proteins reduce the activity of angiotensin converting enzyme (ACE), thereby reducing hypertension. All of this spells out a great weight loss grain.[75]

80. **Add oatmeal** – Oatmeal is a dynamo when it comes to weight loss, offering several benefits to those who are trying to take off a few pounds. Oatmeal is one of the most filling foods that you can eat for breakfast, according to Dr. Mary Ellen Camire, Ph.D., professor of food science and nutrition at the University of Maine. Not only does it beat out doughnuts and white bread in satiety rankings, but it also trumps eggs and high-bran cereal. Research from the University of Maryland Medical Center also counts oats as part of a healthy weight-loss diet. Include oatmeal into your diet daily, and your scale may show a difference.[76]

81. **Add kefir** – Kefir is a thick drink made by fermenting milk with kefir grains composed of lactic acid bacteria, yeast, and polysaccharides. The grains culture the milk, infusing it with healthy organisms. These types of healthy bacteria or probiotics are not available in yogurt. They help to support the digestive system and prevent the growth of harmful bacteria in the intestines. *Men's Health,* Editor in

Chief, David Zincenko recently touted a product called kefir as one of his favorite six essential flat belly foods. But unless you are from Russia or really pay attention when visiting the yogurt aisle at the grocery store, chances are, you've never heard of this 2,000-year-old nutritional rock star. Besides containing less sugar and more protein than conventional yogurt, kefir is packed with probiotics which are bacteria that help maintain the natural balance of organisms in the intestines. Most yogurts contain 1 or 2 strains, and kefir contains a whopping 10 strains.[77]

Some other yogurt versus kefir differences that highlight kefir's nutritional powerhouse status:
- **Calories:** 100 (6 oz. of Yoplait) versus 160 (8 oz. of Lifeway kefir).
- **Fiber:** 0 grams versus 3 grams.
- **Protein:** 5 grams versus 11 grams.
- **Calcium:** 20% Daily Value versus 30%.

82. **Add beans** – A cup of black beans packs a whopping 15 grams of satisfying protein and doesn't contain any of the saturated fat found in other protein sources, like red meat. According to WebMD, bean eaters weigh, on average, 7 pounds less and had slimmer waists than their bean-avoiding counterparts – yet they consumed 199 calories more per day if they were adults and an incredible 335 calories more if they were teenagers.

Dawn Jackson Blatner, RD, a registered dietitian at Northwestern Memorial Hospital's Wellness Institute in Chicago says that beans have something else that meat lacks: phytochemicals, compounds found only in plants. Beans are high in antioxidants, a class of phytochemicals that incapacitate cell-damaging free radicals in the body. Free radicals have been implicated in everything from cancer and aging to neurodegenerative diseases like Parkinson's and Alzheimer's.[78]

83. Add berries – According to Joy Bauer, one of the nation's leading health authorities and the nutrition and health expert for NBC's TODAY show, 'berries are "juicy foods," which means they contain mostly water. Juicy foods are great for losing weight because they fill you up quickly, since their high water content bumps up the volume while driving down the calories. Berries also contain fiber and folate. Fiber aids in weight loss and helps lower cholesterol and blood pressure. Folate may protect against cardiovascular disease and age-related memory loss, and since folate contributes to the production of serotonin, it may also help to ward off depression and improve your mood.'[79]

84. Add chili peppers and ginger – According to an article in the N.Y. Times, capsaicin – the compound that gives these spices their kick – gives a spike to the heat generation in your body which helps to burn more calories after a meal. In studies, capsaicin has shown to increase an average person's metabolism about 8% over their normal rate.[80]

85. Add black pepper – As well as relieving heartburn symptoms and indigestion, pepper grinds away fats, according to research published in the journal *Nutrition Today*. Piperine, the active chemical in black pepper, puts your nervous system in active mode which boosts the body's metabolic process resulting in more calories being burned.[81]

CHAPTER 6
DROP

Don't rely on the food manufacturers to only provide nutritious food for you. They are in it for the money. If salt, sugar, and fat are what people will buy, then they will create laboratory food that meets the demands at the cheapest cost. It's up to you to be in charge of your health, and that means being diligent to read labels and recognize the ingredients that a product is cheaply or chemically made. Here are some ingredients that rank the highest on my gross-me-out-don't-ever-eat list. If you have them in your pantry, just throw them out.

86. **High fructose corn syrup** – High fructose corn syrup (HFCS) is a highly refined artificial sweetener, which has become the number one source of calories in America. It is found in almost all processed foods. HFCS packs on the pounds faster than any other ingredient, increases your LDL ("bad") cholesterol levels, and contributes to the development of diabetes and tissue damage, among other harmful effects.[82]

A Princeton University research team has demonstrated that all sweeteners are not equal when it comes to weight gain: Rats with access to high-fructose corn syrup gained significantly more weight than those with access to table sugar, even when their overall caloric intake was the same. In addition to causing significant weight gain in lab animals, long-term consumption of high-fructose corn syrup also led to abnormal increases in body fat, especially in the abdomen, and a rise in circulating blood fats called triglycerides. The researchers say the work sheds light on the factors contributing to obesity trends in the United States.[83]

In another study, over the course of 6 or 7 months, both male and female rats with access to HFCS gained significantly more body weight than control groups. This increase in body weight with HFCS was accompanied by an increase in adipose fat, notably in the abdominal region, and elevated circulating triglyceride levels. Translated to humans, these results suggest that excessive consumption of HFCS may contribute to the incidence of obesity.[84]

87. **Artificial sweeteners** – Aspartame, more popularly known as Nutrasweet and Equal, is found in foods labeled "diet" or "sugar-free." They disrupt the body's ability to regulate blood sugar, causing metabolic changes that trigger diabetes. Dr. Eran Elinav, physician and immunologist at the Weizmann Institute of Science in Israel said, "Artificial sweeteners are responsible for the onset of the very same condition that we often aim to prevent by consuming sweeteners instead of sugar." In research published in the journal *Nature,* the study found that zero-calorie sweeteners such as saccharin, sucralose, and aspartame can alter the population of bacteria in the gut and trigger high blood glucose levels which can lead to diabetes. Scientists ran tests on 381 people who consumed the most artificial sweeteners and found that these people had different gut microbes and were generally heavier and more glucose intolerant than the rest. Aspartame is believed to be carcinogenic and accounts for more reports of adverse reactions than all other foods and food additives combined. Aspartame is also a neurotoxin known to erode intelligence and affect short-term memory. The components of this toxic sweetener may lead to a wide variety of ailments including brain tumors,

lymphoma, diabetes, multiple sclerosis, Parkinson's, Alzheimer's, fibromyalgia, and chronic fatigue, as well as emotional disorders like depression and anxiety attacks, dizziness, headaches, nausea, mental confusion, migraines and seizures.[85]

88. Endocrine disrupters – According to the National Institute of Environmental Health Sciences, endocrine disruptors are chemicals that may interfere with the body's endocrine system and produce adverse developmental, reproductive, neurological, and immune effects in both humans and wildlife. A wide range of substances, both natural and man-made, are thought to cause endocrine disruption, including pharmaceuticals, dioxin and dioxin-like compounds, polychlorinated biphenyls, DDT and other pesticides, and plasticizers such as bisphenol A (BPA). Endocrine disruptors may be found in many everyday products– including plastic bottles, metal food cans, detergents, flame retardants, food, toys, cosmetics, and pesticides. So what's a mom to do? Substitute stainless steel water bottles for plastic bottles, glass storage containers for plastic ones, frozen food for canned food where possible or look for 'BPA free' on the can label. Many soups come in boxes which are also better than canned goods. Look for clothing without flame retardants. Read your cosmetic labels. Buy organic fruits and vegetables, especially if you eat the skin.[86]

89. Nitrates and sulfates – Commonly found in packaged meats, wine, and other processed foods, these flavor enhancers do nothing but expand your waistline. They attack your digestive system, making it difficult for your body to absorb nutrients from even healthy food.[87]

According to a recent European study, eating lots of meat may be contributing to weight gain. Even among people eating roughly the same overall calories, those that eat meat are more likely to weigh more than those who do not. Over 400,000 Europeans from ten different countries participated in the study, which was published in the *American Journal of Clinical Nutrition*. Participants filled out diet and lifestyle questionnaires and were weighed both at the start of the study, and at five years later. Overall, meat consumption was found to be linked to weight gain in both men and women. The worst meat offender for weight gain is processed meat, which may be due to the nitrites, nitrates, and other chemical preservatives they contain.[88]

90. **Soda** – According to the Harvard School of Public Health, rising consumption of sugary drinks has been a major contributor to the obesity epidemic. A typical 20-ounce soda contains 15 to 18 teaspoons of sugar and upwards of 240 calories. A 64-ounce fountain cola drink could have up to 700 calories. People who drink this "liquid candy" do not feel as full as if they had eaten the same calories from solid food and do not compensate by eating less. A 20-year study on 120,000 men and women found that people who increased their sugary drink consumption by one 12-ounce serving per day gained more weight over time – on average, an extra pound every 4 years – than people who did not change their intake. Other studies have found a significant link between sugary drink consumption and weight gain in children. One study found that for each additional 12-ounce soda children consumed each day, the odds of becoming obese increased by 60% during 1½ years of follow-up. People who consume sugary drinks regularly – 1 to 2 cans a day or more – have a 26% greater risk of developing type 2 diabetes than people who rarely have such drinks. Risks are even higher in young adults and Asians.[89]

91. White sugar – Eating less sugar is linked with weight loss, and eating more is linked with weight gain, according to a new review of published studies in New Zealand.

The review lends support to the idea that advising people to limit the sugar in their diets may help to lessen excess weight and obesity, the New Zealand researchers conclude.

"The really interesting finding is that increasing and decreasing sugar had virtually identical results [on weight], in the opposite direction of course," says researcher Jim Mann, DM, Ph.D., professor of human nutrition and medicine at the University of Otago.

Mann and his team analyzed the results of 30 clinical trials and 38 other studies.[90]

92. Monosodium glutamate (MSG) – MSG is an amino acid used as a flavor enhancer in soups, salad dressings, chips, frozen entrees, and many restaurant foods. Known as an excitotoxin, MSG is a substance which overexcites cells to the point of damage or death. Studies show that regular consumption of it may result in adverse side effects which include depression, disorientation, eye damage, fatigue, headaches, and obesity. MSG affects the neurological pathways of the brain and disengages the function that tells you when you are full which explains the effects of weight gain.[91]

According to a study by the *American Journal of Clinical Nutrition*, MSG is positively associated with overweight development among healthy adults. After analyzing MSG intake and weight gain among more than 10,000 Chinese adults, researchers found that those who ate the most MSG were about 30 percent more likely to become overweight than those who ate the least. The researchers speculated that the hormone leptin might be involved in the weight gain, as those who consumed more MSG also produced more leptin.[92]

CHAPTER 7
THE NEXT LEVEL

Sometimes it doesn't have to do with what you eat; it has to do with lifestyle, body type, metabolic reactions and your own bio-individuality. Here are a few tips that will give you the edge you need to live the healthy life you were meant to live and take it to the next level.

93. **Keep a food journal** – Women who do will lose 6 pounds more on average according to the *Journal of the Academy of Nutrition and Dietetics.*[93]

94. **Get 6 to 8 hours of sleep a night** – Without it, the appetite hormone ghrelin increase, which could result in weight gain, according to Manuel Villacorta RD, author of *Eating Free*. In the Wisconsin Sleep Cohort Study, 1,024 volunteers underwent nocturnal polysomnography and reported on their sleep habits through questionnaires and sleep diaries. During the study, fasting blood samples were evaluated for serum leptin and ghrelin (two key opposing hormones in appetite regulation). Participants with short sleep had reduced leptin and elevated ghrelin. These differences in leptin and ghrelin are likely to increase appetite, possibly explaining the increased BMI observed with short sleep duration. In Western societies, where chronic sleep restriction is common, and food is widely available, changes in appetite regulatory hormones with sleep curtailment may contribute to obesity.[94]

95. **Get checked for food allergies** – Do you typically have achy joints, headaches or fatigue? You could

have a food allergy and not even know it. Eating food you're allergic to doesn't only cause weight gain, it causes inflammation, which can lead to worse diseases down the road. Dr. Hyman, author of the *10 Day Detox Diet* states, "we already know that inflammation from any cause – bacteria, food, a high-sugar, high-fat diet – will produce insulin resistance, leading to higher insulin levels. And since insulin is a fat storage hormone, you store more fat – mostly around the belly."

The authors of two studies that he discusses at www.drhyman.com go on to say that we should consider the elimination of IgG food allergens as a way of treating obesity and preventing heart disease. That means you don't limit calories, just foods that cause allergies that in turn cause inflammation. This study draws a remarkable link that has received little attention by conventional medicine.[95]

96. **Get a nutrients blood panel check** – Metabolism depends on a balanced body. The body is intricately interwoven with hundreds of metabolic factors, throw one off and it's like a house of cards… it all comes tumbling down. The average American diet is rather unbalanced to begin with: heavy on animal foods, processed foods, fried foods, and sweets and light on fruits, vegetables, and whole grains. In his book, *Cracking the Metabolic Code*, James LaValle, a pharmacist and naturopathic physician based in Cincinnati, OH, says that nutrient imbalances of various sorts can lead to weight gain, and conversely, how improving nutrient balance can facilitate weight loss. Likewise, being low in vitamin D, magnesium, or iron can compromise your immune system, sap your energy levels, or alter your metabolism in ways that make it harder to take healthy-lifestyle steps. "You may compensate for low energy with caffeine, sweets, and simple carbs,"

says Dr. Hedaya, "Or find that you feel too run down or weak to exercise."[96]

97. **Check your blood type** – Some people can tolerate dairy. But a significant number of people, unsuspectingly are sensitive to it and don't even know it. Food sensitivities if unchecked can lead to inflammation, which in turn, can lead to weight gain and other chronic diseases. For example, according to the book, *The Blood Type Diet*, if you are blood type O, which is the majority of American people as it is the oldest blood type known, then eating dairy and wheat will cause inflammation fat. Initial weight loss can be achieved by cutting out the foods that cause inflammation for your blood type.[97] See Blood Types Food Chart here:
http://www.soulcraft.co/info/food_chart.htm

98. **Don't go gluten-free without a plan** – Going gluten free is a hot topic in the diet world today, but living gluten-free can make you fat, says Dr. Arthur Agatston medical director of wellness and prevention for Baptist Health South Florida and author of the book, *The South Beach Diet Gluten Solution*. Some people who go off gluten to lose weight end up gaining weight instead. That's because they consume gluten-free packaged products that are often just as high in saturated fat, sugar and sodium as other junk food, and these products often contain high-glycemic refined ingredients like white rice flour or fillers like potato starch that can affect your blood sugar and trigger cravings.[98]

99. **Take a detox bath 2 times per week** – Dr. Oz recommends a detox bath in his 2-week rapid weight loss plan. Simply add 2 cups of Epsom salts and 1 cup of baking soda to your tub. This will carry toxins out of your skin and body and create

alkalinity in your body. Acidity is connected to inflammation, fat, and disease.[99]

100. Wear a pedometer – to track your steps. If you aren't getting 10,000 steps a day, then you know you aren't getting enough. If you're one of those people who believe that only vigorous exercise counts toward fitness, you'd better think again, says Ross Andersen, Ph.D., associate professor of medicine at Johns Hopkins School of Medicine in Baltimore. The research that Dr. Andersen and others have done proves that increasing your everyday activities – walking the dog and just getting up more often – can make a big difference. *Prevention* magazine conducted their own study and put a group of overweight people on a walking pedometer program to lose weight. Based on the number of steps they normally took, they divided them into two groups. Those who were most inactive had a goal of 10,000 steps, while those who were more active had a goal of 18,000 steps. After just 8 weeks, they saw improvements in weight, body fat, cholesterol, and fitness.[100]

CONCLUSION

Congratulations!

You've learned new ways to get to your weight loss goal without dieting.

Once you get in the habit of choosing real food over processed, low nutrient food, you will see your body changing, your energy soaring, your mood lifting and your sleep habits improving. Counting calories is the way our parents used to lose weight; it's old school. Real food is IN and here to stay. It's a way of life that will never go out of style.

For more information and free health tips, recipes, guide, and videos, visit me at www.groovybeets.com.

To groovy health,

Leann

BIBLIOGRAPHY

[1] "8 Ways to Burn Calories and Fight Fat." WebMD. Accessed September 20, 2014. http://www.webmd.com/diet/features/8-ways-to-burn-calories-and-fight-fat?page=2

[2] "National Center for Biotechnology Information. Accessed September 21, 2014. http://www.ncbi.nlm.nih.gov/pubmed/7369170

[3] "Is Eight Enough? U Researcher Says Drink Up and Tells Why." Is Eight Enough? U Researcher Says Drink Up and Tells Why. Accessed September 21, 2014. http://healthcare.utah.edu/publicaffairs/news/archive/2003/new s_74.php.

[4] "Dr. Joel Fuhrman's Food Pyramid." The Dr. Oz Show. Accessed September 21, 2014. http://www.doctoroz.com/videos/dr-joel-fuhrmans-food-pyramid

[5] "Protein: Your Secret Weight-Loss Weapon." Womenshealthmag.com. Accessed September 21, 2014. http://www.womenshealthmag.com/weight-loss/protein-weight-loss

[6] "American Journal of Epidemiology." Association between Eating Patterns and Obesity in a Free-living US Adult Population. Accessed September 21, 2014. http://aje.oxfordjournals.org/content/158/1/85.full

[7] Freston, Kathy. "Day 5: Put a Little Flax on It." The Huffington Post. April 20, 2012. Accessed September 21, 2014. http://www.huffingtonpost.com/kathy-freston/lean-challenge_b_1432764.html

[8] "Result Filters." National Center for Biotechnology Information. Accessed September 21, 2014. http://www.ncbi.nlm.nih.gov/pubmed/22008705 "Download PDFs." Salad and Satiety. The Effect of Timing of Salad Consumption on Meal Energy Intake. Accessed September 21, 2014. http://www.sciencedirect.com/science/article/pii/S01956663110 0599X

[9] "It's All About Eating Right." Academy of Nutrition and Dietetics. Accessed September 21, 2014. http://www.eatright.org/public

[10] "Bob Harper - Skinny Rule #7-no Carbs after Lunch-is One Of... | Facebook." Bob Harper - Skinny Rule #7-no Carbs after Lunch-is One Of... | Facebook. Accessed September 21, 2014. https://www.facebook.com/mytrainerbob/posts/1015089300182 5205

[11] "Restricting Night-time Eating Reduces Daily Energy Intake in Healthy Young Men: A Short-term Cross-over Study." Cambridge Journals Online. Accessed September 21, 2014. http://journals.cambridge.org/action/displayAbstract%3Bjsessioni d%3DC8C6F12F16736CD33711478E3A66CC.journals?aid=9080 129&fileId=S0007114513001359

[12] "Online Library | Articles | G-BOMBS: Greens, Beans, Onions, Mushrooms, Berries, and Seeds | DrFuhrman.com." Online Library | Articles | G-BOMBS: Greens, Beans, Onions, Mushrooms, Berries, and Seeds | DrFuhrman.com. Accessed September 21, 2014. https://www.drfuhrman.com/library/gbombs.aspx

[13] "Weight Loss Plan." Medifast. Accessed September 21, 2014. http://www.medifast1.com/weight_loss_plan/index.jsp

[14] Hasbrouck, Stephanie. "What Is 'clean Eating?' Tips from Expert Tosca Reno." CNN. January 01, 1970. Accessed September 21, 2014. http://www.cnn.com/2012/09/19/health/tosca-reno-clean-eating/

[15] "7 Fermented Foods You Should Be Eating." Prevention. Accessed September 21, 2014. http://www.prevention.com/food/healthy-eating-tips/7-fermented-foods-you-should-be-eating

[16] "Looking to Boost Your Metabolism? Make Sure You Do This." The Huffington Post. Accessed September 21, 2014. http://www.huffingtonpost.ca/dr-john-dempster/boosting-metabolism_b_4729801.html

[17] "Anti-Inflammatory Diet & Pyramid." Anti-Inflammatory Diet. Accessed September 21, 2014. http://www.drweil.com/drw/u/ART02012/anti-inflammatory-diet

[18] "Dr. Pickering: Why Food Combining Matters." Mercola.com. Accessed September 21, 2014. http://articles.mercola.com/sites/articles/archive/2013/10/27/food-combining.aspx

[19] "Journal of Nutrition." Impact of Peanuts and Tree Nuts on Body Weight and Healthy Weight Loss in Adults. Accessed September 21, 2014. http://jn.nutrition.org/content/138/9/1741S.full

[20] "National Institute of Environmental Health Sciences." Endocrine Disruptors. Accessed September 21, 2014. http://www.niehs.nih.gov/health/topics/agents/endocrine

[21] "Quick Ways to Lose Lower Belly Fat." LIVESTRONG.COM. March 27, 2011. Accessed September 21, 2014. http://www.livestrong.com/article/135435-quick-ways-lose-lower-belly-fat/

[22] "THE SKINNY TRUTHS." THE SKINNY How I Went from a Size 10 to a 2 in 4 Months by Eating More and Exercising Less. Accessed September 22, 2014. http://www.theskinny.us.com/the-skinny-truths

[23] "Iodine Deficiency." American Thyroid Association. Accessed September 22, 2014. http://www.thyroid.org/iodine-deficiency/ "Thyroid and Weight." American Thyroid Association. Accessed September 22, 2014. http://www.thyroid.org/weight-loss-and-thyroid/

[24] "The American Journal of Clinical Nutrition." Hidden Vegetables: An Effective Strategy to Reduce Energy Intake and Increase Vegetable Intake in Adults. Accessed September 23, 2014. http://ajcn.nutrition.org/content/93/4/756.abstract?sid=8798feae-7f22-4d9a-bddf-c91bb90e9c66

[25] "Result Filters." National Center for Biotechnology Information. Accessed September 23, 2014. http://www.ncbi.nlm.nih.gov/pubmed/14649970

[26] "Result Filters." National Center for Biotechnology Information. Accessed September 21, 2014. http://www.ncbi.nlm.nih.gov/pubmed/18800884

http://thescienceofeating.com/vegetables/benefits-of-chlorella/)

[27] "Can Probiotics Help You Lose Weight?" Womenshealthmag.com. Accessed September 21, 2014. http://www.womenshealthmag.com/weight-loss/probiotics

[28] "Fats and Cholesterol: Out with the Bad, In with the Good." The Nutrition Source. Accessed September 21, 2014. http://www.hsph.harvard.edu/nutritionsource/fats-full-story/

[29] "Multivitamins and Mineral Therapy for Obesity, Weight Control, Weight Loss, Strategies for Weight Loss, Dieting, Holisticonline.com." Multivitamins and Mineral Therapy for Obesity, Weight Control, Weight Loss, Strategies for Weight Loss, Dieting, Holisticonline.com. Accessed September 21, 2014. http://holisticonline.com/remedies/weight/weight_multiminerals-therapy-for-obesity.htm

[30] "Vitamin D Helps or Hinders Weight Management." Mercola.com. Accessed September 21, 2014. http://articles.mercola.com/sites/articles/archive/2012/08/21/vitamin-d-on-weight-management.aspx

[31] "The Best Vitamins That Aid in Weight Loss." NaturalNews. Accessed September 21, 2014. http://www.naturalnews.com/041663_b_vitamins_nutritional_supplements_weight_loss.html

[32] "Result Filters." National Center for Biotechnology Information. Accessed September 21, 2014. http://www.ncbi.nlm.nih.gov/pubmed/15930480

[33] Perricone, Dr. Nicholas. "The Top 10 Weight Loss Supplements." The Huffington Post. July 08, 2009. Accessed September 21, 2014. http://www.huffingtonpost.com/dr-nicholas-perricone/the-top-10-weight-loss-su_b_227618.html

[34] "L-Glutamine and Weight Loss." LIVESTRONG.COM. August 16, 2013. Accessed September 21, 2014. http://www.livestrong.com/article/232707-l-glutamine-and-weight-loss/

[35] "Vanadium Helps With Weight Loss and Blood Sugar Control | Uber Articles." Uber Articles RSS. Accessed September 21, 2014. http://uberarticles.com/food-and-drink/nutrition/decrease-

blood-sugar-and-weight-with-vanadium/

[36] "7 Belly Blasters That Really Work!" The Dr. Oz Show. Accessed September 21, 2014. http://www.doctoroz.com/videos/7-belly-blasters-really-work

[37] "Result Filters." National Center for Biotechnology Information. Accessed September 21, 2014. http://www.ncbi.nlm.nih.gov/pubmed/19437058

[38] "Can African Mango Be an Effective Weight Loss Aid?" About. Accessed September 21, 2014. http://altmedicine.about.com/od/weight_Loss/a/African-Mango-For-Weight-Loss.htm

[39] Kilham, Chris. "Coffee: An Effective Weight Loss Tool." Fox News. March 21, 2012. Accessed September 21, 2014. http://www.foxnews.com/health/2012/03/21/coffee-effective-weight-loss-tool/

[40] "Lipoic Acid Reverses Mitochondrial Decay â€" Life Extension." LifeExtension.com. Accessed September 21, 2014. http://www.lef.org/magazine/mag2011/aug2011_Lipoic-Acid-Reverses-Mitochondrial-Decay_01.htm

[41] "Why Maitake Is a Must-Have: Immune System and Weight Loss Benefits." Perricone MDs Best Anti Aging Skin Care Products Why Maitake Is a MustHave Immune System and Weight Loss Benefits Comments. Accessed September 21, 2014. http://blog.perriconemd.com/why-maitake-is-a-must-have-immune-system-and-weight-loss-benefits/#2

[42] "Is Organic Dairy Milk the Healthy Option or Are We Being Sold down the River?" Viva! Health. Accessed September 21, 2014. http://www.vegetarian.org.uk/features/display.php?pid=16

[43] "The Advantages of Coconut Yogurt." LIVESTRONG.COM. May 03, 2014. Accessed September 21, 2014. http://www.livestrong.com/article/447127-the-advantages-of-coconut-yogurt/
"Medium Chain Triglycerides (MCTs)." Nutrition Review RSS. Accessed September 21, 2014. http://nutritionreview.org/2013/04/medium-chain-triglycerides-mcts/

[44] "Cheese." - Best Superfoods for Weight Loss. Accessed September 21, 2014.
http://www.health.com/health/gallery/0%2C%2C20475957_23%2C00.html

[45] "Result Filters." National Center for Biotechnology Information. Accessed September 21, 2014.
http://www.ncbi.nlm.nih.gov/pubmed/22474577

[46] "Can Eating Salt Prevent Weight Loss?" LIVESTRONG.COM. February 07, 2014. Accessed September 21, 2014.
http://www.livestrong.com/article/293500-does-salt-stop-weight-loss/

[47] "Changes in Diet and Lifestyle and Long-Term Weight Gain in Women and Men — NEJM." New England Journal of Medicine. Accessed September 21, 2014.
http://www.nejm.org/doi/full/10.1056/NEJMoa1014296#t=abstract

[48] "Journal of Nutrition & Food Sciences." Chickpeas and Hummus Are Associated with Better Nutrient Intake, Diet Quality, and Levels of Some Cardiovascular Risk Factors: National Health and Nutrition Examination Survey 2003-2010. Accessed September 21, 2014.
http://omicsonline.org/nutrition-food-sciences-abstract.php?abstract_id=22385

[49] "Whole Grain Fact Sheet." (EUFIC). Accessed September 21, 2014.
http://www.eufic.org/article/en/expid/Whole-grain-Fact-Sheet/

[50] "How to Substitute Applesauce for Oil." EHow. October 06, 2008. Accessed September 22, 2014.
http://www.ehow.com/how_4535777_substitute-applesauce-oil.html

[51] "Top 50 Summer Diet Foods for Weight Loss." Shape Magazine. Accessed September 22, 2014. http://www.shape.com/weight-loss/food-weight-loss/top-50-summer-diet-foods-weight-loss/slide/22

[52] "Consumer Reports: Bison Vs. Beef Burgers - CBS Pittsburgh." CBS Pittsburgh. Accessed September 22, 2014.
http://pittsburgh.cbslocal.com/2013/07/04/consumer-reports-bison-vs-beef-burgers/

[53] "Top Secret Weight-Loss Food: Mushrooms." The Dr. Oz Show. Accessed September 22, 2014. http://www.doctoroz.com/article/top-secret-weight-loss-food-mushrooms
"Meat That Is Good for Weight Loss." LIVESTRONG.COM. March 19, 2014. Accessed September 22, 2014. http://www.livestrong.com/article/478710-meat-that-is-good-for-weight-loss/

[54] "Tennessee Today." Yogurt Increases Fat Loss, UT Study Shows. Accessed September 22, 2014. http://tntoday.utk.edu/2003/04/14/yogurt-increases-fat-loss-ut-study-shows/

[55] "5 Facts About Quinoa Nutrition and Cooking Quinoa (Page 3)." 5 Facts About Quinoa Nutrition and Cooking Quinoa (Page 3). Accessed September 22, 2014. http://www.eatingwell.com/healthy_cooking/healthy_cooking_101_basics_techniques/5_facts_about_quinoa_nutrition_and_cooking_quinoa?page=3

[56] "The Amazing Wonder of Coconut Butter (And How to Actually Use It)." 12 Minute Athlete. Accessed September 22, 2014. http://www.12minuteathlete.com/coconut-butter/

[57] Nickle, Melissa, and Pamela Pehrsson. "USDA Updates Nutrient Values for Fast Food Pizza." *Procedia Food Science* 2 (2013): 87-92. doi:10.1016/j.profoo.2013.04.014. http://www.ars.usda.gov/SP2UserFiles/Place/12354500/Articles/ProcediaFS2_87-92.pdf

[58] "Sugar in Peanut Butter." Nutrition Action. Accessed September 22, 2014. http://www.nutritionaction.com/daily/sugar-in-food/sugar-in-peanut-butter/

[59] "The American Journal of Clinical Nutrition." The Effects of a Whole Grain–enriched Hypocaloric Diet on Cardiovascular Disease Risk Factors in Men and Women with Metabolic Syndrome. Accessed September 22, 2014. http://ajcn.nutrition.org/content/87/1/79.abstract

[60] Wise, Abigail. "Ask A Scientist: Is Honey Healthier Than Sugar?" The Huffington Post. June 09, 2014. Accessed September 22, 2014. http://www.huffingtonpost.com/2014/06/09/healthy-sugar-honey_n_5445024.html

[61] "Organic Gluten-Free Coconut Flour." Mercola.com. Accessed September 22, 2014. http://products.mercola.com/coconut-flour/

[62] Bratskeir, Kate. "How To Make The Vegan Ice Cream That Everyone's Eating Right Now." The Huffington Post. August 12, 2014. Accessed September 22, 2014. http://www.huffingtonpost.com/2014/08/12/vegan-ice-cream-recipe-no-dairy-no-problem_n_5666795.html

[63] "15 Secret Weight-loss Solutions." Men's Health. Accessed September 22, 2014. http://www.menshealth.co.uk/lose-weight/fast-tips/15-secret-weight-loss-solution-2

[64] "Can Eating Squash Help Me Lose Weight?" Live Well. Accessed September 22, 2014. http://livewell.jillianmichaels.com/can-eating-squash-lose-weight-5505.html

[65] Lanou, Amy Joy, and Barbara Svenson. "Abstract." National Center for Biotechnology Information. December 20, 2010. Accessed September 22, 2014. http://www.ncbi.nlm.nih.gov/pmc/articles/PMC3048091/

[66] "Conditions We Diagnose and Treat." Dr. Robynne Chutkan. Accessed September 22, 2014. http://www.robynnechutkan.com/content/conditions-we-diagnose-and-treat

[67] "HowStuffWorks "How Vinegar Affects Digestion"" HowStuffWorks. Accessed September 22, 2014. http://health.howstuffworks.com/wellness/food-nutrition/facts/the-health-benefits-of-vinegar3.htm

[68] "Result Filters." National Center for Biotechnology Information. Accessed September 22, 2014. http://www.ncbi.nlm.nih.gov/pubmed/21442412

[69] Elaine Magee, MPH, RDWebMD Weight Loss Clinic - Expert Column. "The Secret of Edamame." WebMD. Accessed September 22, 2014. http://www.webmd.com/diet/features/the-secret-of-edamame

[70] "Prebiotics: Secret Ingredient That Helps Burn Belly Fat March 27 2014." The LynFit Shop. Accessed September 22, 2014. http://lynfit.com/blogs/news/13144977-prebiotics-secret-

ingredient-that-helps-burn-belly-fat

[71] Freston, Kathy. "An Apple a Day Melts the Pounds Away!" The Huffington Post. April 12, 2012. Accessed September 22, 2014. http://www.huffingtonpost.com/kathy-freston/apples-health_b_1418993.html

[72] "Result Filters." National Center for Biotechnology Information. Accessed September 22, 2014. http://www.ncbi.nlm.nih.gov/pubmed/16579728

[73] MailOnline, Lizzie Parry for. "Spinach Helps You Lose Weight by Curbing Cravings for Sweet Treats and Junk Food." Mail Online. September 03, 2014. Accessed September 22, 2014. http://www.dailymail.co.uk/health/article-2742026/Spinach-extract-boosts-weight-loss-50-curbing-cravings-sweet-treats-junk-food.html#ixzz3Cq3CsjOR

[74] "Anti Estrogenic Diet." Anti Estrogenic Diet. Accessed September 22, 2014. http://www.everydiet.org/diet/anti-estrogenic-diet

[75] "Dr. Perricone's No. 5 Superfood: Buckwheat." Oprah.com. Accessed September 22, 2014. http://www.oprah.com/health/Buckwheat-Dr-Perricones-No-5-Superfood

[76] "Hypercholesterolemia." University of Maryland Medical Center. Accessed September 22, 2014. http://umm.edu/health/medical/altmed/condition/hypercholesterolemia

[77] "Benefits Of Kefir." The Science Of Eating. Accessed September 22, 2014. http://thescienceofeating.com/proteins/benefits-of-kefir/ Goldman, Leslie. "The Flat Belly Food You Don't Know About: Kefir." The Huffington Post. August 04, 2009. Accessed September 22, 2014. http://www.huffingtonpost.com/leslie-goldman/the-flat-belly-food-you-d_b_250273.html

[78] Jenny Stamos KovacsWebMD the Magazine - Feature. "Beans: Protein-Rich Superfoods." WebMD. Accessed September 22, 2014. http://www.webmd.com/diet/features/beans-protein-rich-superfoods

"Black Beans." - Best Superfoods for Weight Loss. Accessed September 22, 2014.

http://www.health.com/health/gallery/0%2C%2C20475957_2%2
C00.html

[79] "Health Benefits of Berries." Www.joybauer.com. Accessed September
21, 2014. http://www.joybauer.com/food-articles/berries

[80] O'connor, Anahad. "REALLY?" The New York Times. November 27, 2006.
Accessed September 21, 2014.
http://www.nytimes.com/2006/11/28/health/nutrition/28real.ht
ml?_r=0

[81] "Black Pepper: Overview of Health Benefits" Nutrition Today.
http://journals.lww.com/nutritiontodayonline/Abstract/2010/010
00/Black_Pepper___Overview_of_Health_Benefits.8.aspx

[82] "Top 10 Food Additives to Avoid." Food Matters. Accessed September 22,
2014. http://foodmatters.tv/articles-1/top-10-food-additives-to-
avoid

[83] Parker, By Hilary. "A Sweet Problem: Princeton Researchers Find That
High-fructose Corn Syrup Prompts Considerably More Weight
Gain." Princeton University. March 22, 2010. Accessed September
22, 2014.
http://www.princeton.edu/main/news/archive/S26/91/22K07/

[84] "Result Filters." National Center for Biotechnology Information. Accessed
September 22, 2014.
http://www.ncbi.nlm.nih.gov/pubmed/20219526

[85] "Top 10 Food Additives to Avoid." Food Matters. Accessed September 22,
2014. http://foodmatters.tv/articles-1/top-10-food-additives-to-
avoid

[86] "Endocrine Disruptors." The Internet Journal of Family Practice 10, no. 1
(2012). doi:10.5580/2c82.
https://www.niehs.nih.gov/health/materials/endocrine_disruptor
s_508.pdf

[87] "Why Food Preservatives Keep You Overweight." Health On A Budget.
Accessed September 22, 2014. http://healthonabudget.com/why-
food-preservatives-keep-you-overweight/

[88] "'Cut down on Meat to Lose Weight'" BBC News. July 22, 2010. Accessed
September 22, 2014. http://www.bbc.co.uk/news/health-

10726414

89 "Sugary Drinks and Obesity Fact Sheet." The Nutrition Source. Accessed
September 22, 2014.
http://www.hsph.harvard.edu/nutritionsource/sugary-drinks-
fact-sheet/

90 Doheny, Kathleen. "Sugar and Excess Weight: Evidence Mounts."
WebMD. Accessed September 22, 2014.
http://www.webmd.com/diet/news/20130114/sugar-excess-
weight

91 "Top 10 Food Additives to Avoid." Food Matters. Accessed September 22,
2014. http://foodmatters.tv/articles-1/top-10-food-additives-to-
avoid

92 "The American Journal of Clinical Nutrition." Consumption of
Monosodium Glutamate in Relation to Incidence of Overweight in
Chinese Adults: China Health and Nutrition Survey (CHNS).
Accessed September 22, 2014.
http://ajcn.nutrition.org/content/93/6/1328.
http://www.reuters.com/article/2011/05/27/us-msg-linked-
weight-gaiidUSTRE74Q5SJ20110527).

93 "Result Filters." National Center for Biotechnology Information. Accessed
September 22, 2014.
http://www.ncbi.nlm.nih.gov/pubmed/22795495

94 "Short Sleep Duration Is Associated with Reduced Leptin, Elevated
Ghrelin, and Increased Body Mass Index." PLOS Medicine.
Accessed September 22, 2014.
http://www.plosmedicine.org/article/info%3Adoi/10.1371/journa
l.pmed.0010062

95 "Are Your Food Allergies Making You Fat? - Dr. Mark Hyman." Dr Mark
Hyman. Accessed September 22, 2014.
http://drhyman.com/blog/2010/04/20/are-your-food-allergies-
making-you-fat/#close

96 "7 Surprise Reasons for Weight Gain." Fox News. November 25, 2011.
Accessed September 22, 2014.
http://www.foxnews.com/health/2011/11/25/7-surprise-
reasons-for-weight-gain/

[97] "Blood Type Diet - Type O - DrLam® - Body. Mind. Nutrition®." Blood Type Diet - Type O - DrLam® - Body. Mind. Nutrition®. Accessed September 22, 2014. http://www.drlam.com/blood_type_diet/blood_o.asp

[98] Agatston, Dr. Arthur, and The Opinions Expressed in This Commentary Are Solely Those of Dr. Arthur Agatston. "Gluten: 5 Things You Need to Know." CNN. January 01, 1970. Accessed September 22, 2014. http://www.cnn.com/2013/04/05/health/gluten-5-things/

[99] "Dr. Oz's 2-Week Rapid Weight-Loss Plan Instructions." The Dr. Oz Show. Accessed September 22, 2014. http://www.doctoroz.com/slideshow/dr-ozs-2-week-rapid-weight-loss-plan-instructions?gallery=true&page=3

[100] "Easy Steps to Shape Up and Slim Down." Prevention. Accessed September 22, 2014. http://www.prevention.com/fitness/fitness-tips/walking-pedometer-program-lose-weight